Running 101
A beginner's guide to running

By Matt Hofbauer

CONTENTS

Section 1 – Your First Steps   Page 1

Section 2 – Nutrition and Hydration   Page 10

Section 3 – Training Types   Page 26

Section 4 – Recovery and Injuries   Page 42

Section 5 – Proper Form   Page 50

Section 6 – Ready for Race Day   Page 58

Section 7 – Bonus Material   Page 67

SECTION 1 - YOUR FIRST STEPS

In this section we will discuss the following:
- Getting started
- Picking a goal
- Making a training plan
- Moving toward your goal
- What progress looks like

GETTING STARTED

When you're getting started, remember that you get out exactly what you put in.

We all had a Day 1. Nobody was born a great runner. We all struggled and continue to struggle every day.

The only difference between the runner who's trained for years, the beginner a couple months in, and someone debating whether to go buy shoes is one thing - time invested.

If you are willing to put in the time, you *can* be a runner. This guide will give you the tools you need to start your journey.

Also remember that a healthy runner is a happy runner. Our focus will be on safe and steady progress.

PICKING A GOAL

What are you trying to accomplish? The first step to success is to figure out what your finish line looks like.

This could be to run your first 5K, increase speed, add distance, lose weight, or maintain a healthy lifestyle.

Whatever it is, your training and ability to succeed will be much more effective with a goal and a plan to get there.

When you progress toward a specific goal, you are more likely to stay on track; when you have a clear plan to follow, you are more likely to get back up again if you do fall.

So, figure out what you want to accomplish and write it down. Physically grab a piece of paper and write down your goal (even if that goal is to maintain your current fitness level).

Next, put it up somewhere you'll see it often, like your bathroom mirror. This note will be a constant reminder that you want to, and can, achieve your goal.

Turning your goal into a physical reminder is the first step in making your future finish line a part of the real world; you can touch it and see it.

You have transformed your goal from a thought in your mind to a part of reality before you've even set out for your first run.

This is the first part of progress: deciding what you are progressing toward. From here, we need to outline a plan and figure out how to get there.

MAKING A TRAINING PLAN

A good training plan will hold you accountable and keep you on track. Steady progression is key. Your plan should also be tailored toward your goal.

There are several different components that can go into a training plan. What you include will depend on what your goal is.

Here are some of the basic building blocks common to training plans. (Some of these may not apply to you depending on your goal.)

RUNNING DAYS – This may seem overly obvious but running days will be the foundation of your plan. You need to have established days that are dedicated to running, especially if you want to run 5+ days per week.

Don't set yourself up for failure by being vague. "I'll run three days a week" may leave you stuck trying to run Friday, Saturday and Sunday because life became hectic early in the week.

WHAT GOES INTO A TRAINING PLAN

Rest days — Equally important to running days are rest days. Again, establishing this time is especially important in plans with 5+ running days. You need prescribed rest in order to properly recover from the physical stress of running.

Cross-training — These are days designated to anything other than running like swimming, strength training, or yoga. To be a good runner you need to be in prime physical health. Cross-training days help you develop an overall better level of fitness, which translates to better running.

Speed, Hills & Long Runs — These are runs tailored to a specific style of training. Incorporating these into your plan will elevate your run days based on your goal. We will discuss each option in a later section.

MOVING TOWARD YOUR GOALS

So, you have your goal and know the basics of a training plan. Now what?

From here I suggest you look at the big picture and divide your goal into manageable chunks.

For example, let's say your goal is to run a half marathon. Your current level of performance is a one mile walk before tiring. Let's also say you have 8 months to get from here to there.

To succeed without setting yourself up for failure, you need a realistic path forward.

Instead of looking at that long 13-mile road in front of you, let's break it down. Let's shoot for a 5K in two months. Use the next three months to reach 10K. Then you have three months left to work up to that half marathon.

Same goal, same time frame, but broken down into smaller chunks with more accomplishments to celebrate.

Continuing with this example, we now have three separate training plans: an 8-week 5K plan, a 12-week 10K plan, and a 12-week half marathon plan. Suddenly, that half marathon doesn't look so far away once we have three manageable pieces and a plan to get there.

Another bonus of starting with smaller races is that you get a taste of race day and all that goes along with it.

If your goal is to maintain where you're at, your training plan can be much simpler. Pick your running days and stick to them. "Monday, Wednesday and Saturday I am going to run a 5K." If this is something you want, write it down and make it happen.

WHAT PROGRESS LOOKS LIKE

When you think of progress, you need to think healthy progress. Those who try to progress too quickly are asking for injury. I am guilty of this myself and have paid for my mistakes > and am reminded by my body every now and then.

So, what does good, healthy progress look like?

There is the unofficial 10% rule that says, "only increase base mileage or volume by 10% per week." The problem with this rule, though, is that our bodies and situations are all vastly different.

If you're a new runner, this might be too aggressive. If you're a veteran runner returning from a short break, 10% might be slower than you need to bounce back to your previous weekly mileage.

New runners should focus on slow, steady progress. This may mean sticking with the same mileage for two or three weeks while your body adjusts. Once you feel comfortable with your mileage, add a couple more and cycle that for a couple weeks.

When building your base as a new runner, don't think about increasing your mileage daily or weekly. Focus on consistent progress over the next few months. Your body is adapting to new stress and needs time.

Pushing hard early on can result in injury, which will hit the reset button on any temporary progress made.

Pay special attention to your body during this base-building phase. Sharp pain or discomfort lasting more than a couple days are two common warning signs that you need to slow down.

Connective tissues and joints are especially troublesome. If you try to push through injury here, recovery time can be especially long.

Remember that a healthy runner is a happy runner. Stay healthy out there!

SECTION 2 — NUTRITION & HYDRATION

In this section we will discuss the following:
- Proper nutrition
- Hydration
- Electrolytes
- Fueling pre-run
- Fueling intra-run
- Fueling post-run

PROPER NUTRITION

Nutrition can help or hurt you as a runner. Since running is high impact and requires a lot of energy, you need to be mindful of how you fuel your body to handle the stress.

Things to include:

- Foods rich in micronutrients - Think fruits and veggies. Micronutrients include all the vitamins and minerals your body needs to function properly. Electrolytes fall into this category, which will help you stay hydrated.

- Protein - Your body is going to be doing a lot of repair work after runs and on rest days, so make sure you have an adequate supply of protein to fuel this process.

- Healthy fats - Some examples are avocados, nuts, and whole eggs. These can help reduce inflammation. Omega-3 fats are especially helpful - try salmon, chia seeds or walnuts.

Things to avoid:

- Refined sugars and high-fructose corn syrup - These can increase inflammation, and even work against the positive effects of omega-3 fats.

- Artificial trans fats - These can significantly increase inflammation. These are often listed as "partially hydrogenated oil" on nutrition labels.

- Alcohol - You knew it was coming. Alcohol in quantities past moderate can be very disruptive to your training and increase inflammation. No one wants to run with a hangover (although it is usually a great cure for one).

Overall, shoot for a balanced diet that will reduce inflammation and provide the fuel you need to maximize your running efforts.

STAYING HYDRATED

Poor hydration can ruin months of training on race day if you're not careful. If neglected, it can require emergency medical attention.

Your body is mostly made of water. That water helps organs function properly, deliver nutrients to cells, remove waste, lubricate joints, and regulate body temperature.

So, in a state of dehydration (depending on severity), you risk your internal organs shutting down, your body overheating, and your body unable to transport nutrients to its cells.

Generally, you can tell how hydrated you are by the color of your urine. The darker the urine, the more dehydrated you are. (However, there are certain medical conditions and foods that can influence the color of urine.)

When running, you will get some pretty loud signals if you're dehydrated.

- Dry mouth - Your body stops or slows the production of saliva.

- Cramping - Cramping in the abdomen is usually caused by dehydration, while cramping in the legs and calves is usually caused by low electrolytes.

- Lack of sweat during physical activity - This is your body's way of trying to conserve water, at the risk of overheating. If this is occurring, you need to start the rehydration process ASAP.

To stay hydrated, continuously drink water throughout the day and during runs, and make sure you are getting enough electrolytes.

Three main causes of dehydration are sweating, vomiting and diarrhea. These can also cause an imbalance in electrolytes as well.

There are also illnesses that cause dehydration or electrolyte imbalance, so consult a medical professional if you think you might be experiencing a severe imbalance.

ELECTROLYTES

Electrolytes are minerals that your body relies on for several different critical functions. They help with nerve signaling, muscle contraction, staying hydrated and balancing your body's PH level.

Most non-runners absorb enough electrolytes through food, but runners who are sweating a lot may need to increase their intake through sports drinks, supplements, or micronutrient-rich food.

When electrolytes are out of balance, you can experience some serious side effects including muscle weakness, confusion, numbness, tingling, fatigue, and in serious cases convulsions.

The electrolytes your body relies on are sodium, chloride, potassium, calcium, magnesium, and phosphate.

The two most critical for runners are sodium and chloride, because these are lost in greater quantities through sweat. (More on these next.)

You will also lose potassium, calcium, and magnesium through sweat, but in lower concentrations. Phosphates are generally lost in non-running ways, such as severely imbalanced nutrition, severe burns, chronic diarrhea, and long-term use of diuretics.

The most important thing to remember about electrolytes is to get them in before your runs. Keep your body in a state of good hydration and keep your electrolyte levels balanced. Again, if you think you are imbalanced or dehydrated, talk to a medical professional.

SODIUM & CHLORIDE

Sodium and chloride help your body regulate water retention. Sodium specifically helps send electrical signals between your brain and muscles via the nervous system.

The two minerals combined make common table salt. (That is why some endurance athletes carry salt tabs or a salt stick, or you might see pickles at race rest stations.)

You need to make sure you're getting enough. People who follow a low-sodium diet should be mindful of how much they run to ensure their sodium levels don't drop too low.
Another cause of low sodium is too much water. Yes, you can drink too much water in relation to electrolyte intake. We lose electrolytes through urine, so drinking excessive amounts of water can flush out electrolytes fast.

Good sources of sodium include dill pickles, tomato juice, sauce and soups, and adding a small amount of table salt to meals.

As with all things running, preparation and maintenance are critical. If you put work in to maintain proper levels of sodium and chloride, you can save yourself a lot of pain and suffering.

POTASSIUM

Potassium is responsible for regulating heartbeat and controlling muscle contraction. It also supports other electrolytes with water retention .

Your body regulates the level of potassium by filtering excess out via the kidneys. You shouldn't lose a lot of potassium through sweat, which means it doesn't have to be a major component in your refueling.

Good sources of potassium include potatoes with skin, plain yogurt, bananas, leafy greens, and salmon.
You should get enough potassium through a well-rounded diet, but if you are prone to low potassium or excessive sweating you may want to supplement.

MAGNESIUM

Magnesium helps the body with biochemical reactions and assists the other electrolytes in nerve and muscle function. It also supports strong bones and a strong immune system.

Good sources of magnesium include leafy greens, nuts, and seeds.

The amount of magnesium in a balanced diet is generally enough to stay in a good range. Since we don't lose magnesium through sweat, this isn't an electrolyte you need to specifically target in your hydration plan.

However, there are medical conditions that can contribute to low magnesium, so consult a medical professional if you think you may be imbalanced.

CALCIUM

Calcium is used by the body to build and maintain healthy bones. About 99% of the calcium in your body is stored in your bones and teeth. Calcium also helps clot blood and assists other electrolytes with muscle contraction.

Dairy is a great source of calcium. Leafy greens and certain vegetables contain it as well but in smaller amounts.

A regular diet should provide enough calcium, and since sweating isn't a primary way of losing large amounts of calcium you shouldn't need to supplement.

However, if you are practicing dietary restrictions that may impact your calcium intake, consider a supplement. Certain medical conditions can contribute to calcium deficiency, so talk with a medical professional if you think you may be low.

PHOSPHATES

Phosphates are similar in function to calcium. They help build and repair bones and teeth and help the nervous system with muscle contractions.

Good sources of phosphates include meat, poultry, fish, and dairy.

Like with most electrolytes, a standard diet should provide enough phosphates. The mineral is lost through urine rather than sweat, so no need to focus on replenishing them during a run. If you have concerns, speak with a medical professional.

FUELING PRE-RUN

Fueling pre-run sets you up for a great run. Take this seriously and your body will thank you. This section will look at same day fueling, rather than the days leading up to a race.

When looking at pre-run fuel, you need to think about what your body will need while on the run.

Generally, our bodies have a hard time utilizing fat for fuel via digestion, so you'll want to focus on carbs pre-run. If you are practicing a low carb diet like keto for weight loss and your runs are shorter in duration carbs pre-run really don't need to be added. If you are practicing low carb as an endurance athlete there are several athletes experimenting with dual fueling carbs and fat that do a partial carb load prior to a longer duration run.

This is also a good time to sneak in electrolytes (salt and potassium especially). You can include protein, but your primary focus should be carbs.

Try to avoid fats and fiber as those sit heavier in your stomach and can be stressful to your digestive system.

Eat a well-rounded meal about three hours before your run, then add something light before you begin.

A pre-run snack is more important for distance runners, those pushing a difficult pace, or those running for more than an hour. If you are running less than an hour, this last-minute snack is less critical.

Remember to stay hydrated. You should be drinking plenty of fluids throughout the day then slowly tapering off before your run so you won't need to stop early to find a bathroom.

A good pre-run meal three hours before might consist of a banana and oatmeal or an English muffin with peanut butter.

A pre-run snack just before race start might be a granola bar or something else your body can easily digest and won't slosh around in your stomach.
Remember to try your pre-run meal and snack prior to race day to find what sits well, then don't change it up last minute.

FUELING INTRA-RUN

Fueling intra-run is helpful for long distance runs of an hour and a half or more. If you are running less than that, this might not be necessary and you can instead focus on pre-nutrition.

Your body has an energy reserve of muscle and liver glycogen. Trial and error will determine how far stored fuel will get you. If you feel a crash that means your body has run out of glycogen and you should consider an intra-run snack.

Fueling during the run can be a bit tricky, especially if you prefer whole foods over running/endurance sport fuels like gels, blocks, and gummies.

Fuel options include:
1. Whole foods - I like things like oatmeal, mashed potatoes, granola bars, or rice cereal added to an electrolyte drink. Some things to consider with whole foods:

- Is it easy to eat? (It shouldn't give you dry mouth, be too chewy, too hard, or fall apart easily.)
- Is it easy to open? (You'll need to open it while running.)
- Is it high in calories? (Focus on carbs and a little protein.)
- Will it stand up to different temperatures? (You don't want it melting in heat or becoming too hard to eat in cold.)

2. Sports fuels (such as race gels, blocks, gummies, etc.) - These work very well and come in a TON of different flavors. The downside is they can be more expensive.

Shoot for 100-300 calories per hour depending on the type of race, overall duration, and intensity.

Remember to stay hydrated during your run. The more you sweat, the more critical this becomes. Think about water and electrolyte replenishment.

Experimentation is your friend here. Find what works and don't try something new on race day.

FUELING POST-RUN

Let's look at what your body is doing during the run to consider what you'll need to replace post-run.

While you run, your body is utilizing stored muscle and liver glycogen (and some fat) for fuel. If you run hard or long enough your body will use up all reserves, leaving you out of stored glycogen.

Your body is also losing water and electrolytes through sweat. Sweating is necessary to regulate temperature, and running produces a lot more heat than resting. Depending on the amount of sweat and intra-run water intake, you may be dehydrated post-run and low on both water and electrolytes.

Lastly, your muscles take a beating when you run (or exercise in general). Your body needs to repair itself, and since protein is a primary building block for this, you need to include it as part of your recovery fuel.

To sum up, a good way to refuel is through a balance of carbs, protein, electrolytes, and fluids.

One example post-run snack would be a banana, protein shake, and an electrolyte sports drink, although you should try to avoid added sugar in shakes and sports drinks.

SECTION 3 – TRAINING TYPES

In this section we will discuss the following:
- Heart rate zone training
- Implementing zone training
- Common training styles
- Speed work
- Hill work
- Long runs

HEART RATE ZONES

If you hate math, hang tight. Understanding these zones will help you be a better runner, because they allow you to tailor your runs based on your objective (building speed versus adding endurance versus a recovery run).

Heart rate zones are specific to each person, and it takes a little math and some trial and error to get them right.
The building blocks include:

Resting Heart Rate (RHR) - Find this by taking your pulse in the morning before you get out of bed. Do this for 5-7 days to get a good average. (Example: 60)

Maximum Heart Rate (MHR) - Find this by subtracting your age from 220. (Example: 195) Keep in mind, this is an average and doesn't consider things like fitness level or genetics.

Heart Rate Reserve (HRR) - Find this by subtracting your resting heart rate from your maximum heart rate. (Example: 135)

You can find an online calculator to do the work for you, or you can use this formula to determine your target heart rate for each zone:
The formula: (x * HRR) + RHR

x represents the percentage of effort that corresponds to the zone you're trying to achieve (those percentages are listed on the next page).

So, to reach zone 2 (which is 60-70% effort) using our example numbers, you would calculate for 60% first:
(.60 * 135) + 60, which equals 141;

then you would calculate for 70%:
(.70 * 135) + 60, which equals 154.5.
So the person in our example would be training in Zone 2 when their heart rate is between 141 and 154.

Zone 1 - 50-60% - recovery run
Zone 2 - 60-70% - fat burning zone
Zone 3 - 70-80% - aerobic zone
Zone 4 - 80-90% - aerobic threshold
Zone 5 - 90-100% - anaerobic zone

Understanding these zones can really elevate your training. Next, we'll look at each zone individually.

ZONE 1

Zone 1 is the lightest or "easiest effort" zone. Each zone gets harder from here. This is your recovery zone, and the pace you should use for warmups and cooldowns.

In this zone, your body works at about 50-60%. This pace should feel like you could go for hours. You should be able to easily carry on a conversation at this pace.

A good indication that you're in this zone is that your body will start to sweat, and you start to feel your muscles warming up.

If you have a recovery run built into your training plan, this is the zone you'll want to target for that. If you are doing any interval training, you most likely will be backing down to a zone 1 recovery pace between repeats. This will allow your body to recover and be fresh for the next working set.

Zone 1 can also help new runners in building an initial base. The lower intensity allows a new runner to get their feet moving without putting too much strain on connective tissue and muscles that aren't used to moving so much.

What zone 1 will not do (or not do very well) is substantially contribute to speed, endurance, or put you into an optimal fat burning state. If you are trying to optimize one of those areas, you're going to have to put in a little more work.

ZONE 2

Of all the zones we'll talk about, pay special attention to Zone 2. It is often overlooked by new runners because of a misperception about running - that you must be out of breath pushing yourself to make progress.

In this zone, your body works at about 60-70%. You should be able to get through short sentences without rushing or breaking for a breath.

The speed of this zone will be specific to the runner. It might even be a walking pace early on. That is OK. As you progress your cardiovascular system will strengthen and you will be able to reach faster speeds while in this zone.

Some benefits of training in Zone 2:

- Burning fat for fuel - Although this won't burn the most calories, your body targets fat for fuel here. It is the optimal zone for your body to start chipping away at fat stores.

- Heart and lung conditioning - In this zone, you are exercising your body's ability to take in oxygen and transport it to the muscle, where it is used to produce fuel. That measurement of oxygen is called your "VO2 max" and we'll discuss that further in a later section.

- Building proper form - You should feel somewhat relaxed in this zone, and able to focus on improving your form. Focus on your foot strike, your cadence, your arm swing, etc. (Proper form will be discussed in Section 5.)

If zone 2 feels like a snail's pace, hang in there. Base building takes time, and zone 2 is the safest way to do it. Think of it as the foundation of your running journey.

I personally train about 75-80% of my weekly miles in this zone when trying to increase base mileage.

ZONE 3

Zone 3 is best described as comfortably difficult.

Your body works at 70-80%. You should be able to speak in short broken sentences, and breathing will be slightly difficult.

Zone 3 training is the upper end of aerobic exercise. Past this point, you will end up out of breath and fatiguing much faster. You can maintain zone 3 for only a moderate amount of time.

Zone 3 is a bit more taxing on the body, so if you incorporate some extended time in this zone, make sure you are stretching, foam rolling, and getting rest.

Some benefits of training in Zone 3:

- Increasing blood flow to the heart and muscles - In zone 3, your body works to increase the number and size of blood vessels. That helps drive more oxygen to the muscles and helps to clear lactic acid and other byproducts from your muscles.

- Burning fat - Your body is still burning a good amount of fat for fuel in this zone. So even if you move from zone 2 into zone 3 during your lower intensity workouts, you're still utilizing stored fat as a fuel source.
  However, the higher you go, the more your body will transition back to preferring carbs (glycogen) as its primary fuel source.

ZONE 4

Here is where the going gets tough.

Zone 4 is almost maximum effort. Your body is working at 80-90% capacity. This is when your body starts utilizing carbs instead of fat for fuel. This is also where your body shifts from aerobic to anaerobic exercise (check the bonus material for a comparison of the two).

Another thing that happens in this zone is your body will start producing lactic acid faster than it is able to filter and remove it. This buildup of lactic acid is what causes a nauseous feeling and ultimately forces you to slow down or stop.

There are benefits to the effort. Training in this zone should increase your tolerance to the lactic acid buildup, and increase your speed and endurance as a result. If you're looking to PR that 5K or increase speed overall, try incorporating this into interval training (more on interval training later).

Again, these higher intensity zones are putting much more stress on your body. As you start to increase intensity, you need to take time to properly recover. Include things like stretching, foam rolling, icing when needed, and (most importantly) rest.

Don't be afraid to take a day off. One day won't offset your training plan, but 2 weeks or 2 months because of an injury will.

Please note, however, that taking an extra day off to recover should be the exception, not the rule. If you find yourself needing to break your plan every other week to add in rest days, you should adjust your plan.

ZONE 5

The final zone. Your maximum effort. You are working at 90-100% effort. This is your "I CAN'T THINK RIGHT NOW" pace. No words, heavy breathing, all out running.

In zone 5, your body works in overdrive to keep up. The lactic acid saturates your body and you will be forced to stop very quickly (usually within a few minutes at best).

If your running journey has just begun, chances are you don't need to train at this intensity. If you have been running for some time and are looking to improve your pace, this may help you.
Training in intervals with zone 5 can really help improve speed. It can also help maintain and even improve your maximum heart rate. There is a saying that goes, "if you want to run faster, you have to run faster."

At this pace, your body will cut you off after a relatively short interval, which is why it is best utilized during high intensity interval training.

Here comes another safety warning. If you are implementing these higher intensity workouts, take a hard look at your recovery plan. Take it seriously. An injury can last over 6 months depending on type and severity, and that's enough to derail an entire running season.

Prevent the injury before it happens and save yourself a whole world of hurt.

IMPLEMENTING HR ZONE TRAINING

Now that you understand the basics and benefits of heart rate zone training, it's time to add them into your training plan.
There are a few ways to do so, but first you should ask whether you are ready to add complexity.

Building a solid foundation is the most important thing for new runners. You should have that base and be comfortable in your current training level before you decide to go faster or farther. Progression is great, but progressing too quickly is a recipe for injury.

If you're reading this saying, "Yes, I am comfortable and ready to start implementing these new techniques," then here we go.

As you start plugging these into your weekly plan, remember that variety will give you the best results. Even if you are training to increase endurance, you shouldn't skip out on all speed work.

Here are three options to implement HR zone training into your plan:
1) High intensity interval day - Warm up in zone 1, push into zones 3-4, recover in zones 1-2, repeat, cool down in zone 1.
2) Threshold run - Sustain zone 3 for the entire working window. Distance and time will depend on your conditioning.
3) Long run - Sustain zone 2 for the entire working window. This will burn fat and increase your base mileage. (Long runs are discussed more in depth later in this section.)

With these three workouts, you should see progress in your endurance and speed. These are generally the most applicable for a new runner to add variety to their training, but there are other variations out there as well.

You don't have to incorporate all three every single week. If you are increasing base mileage, you might have all zone 2 run days except for 1. That odd day could alternate every other week between speed and hills (discussed below). If you aren't interested in increasing mileage, sub the long run out for a zone 2 run at your target distance. There is no set way to achieve a running goal that will work for 100% of the population. Our bodies are all just too different. So experiment and find what works best for you.

COMMON TRAINING STYLES

Let's look at three common training styles then we'll drill down on each.

1) Speed work - This style will help improve your running economy, meaning your body's ability to transport and use oxygen (otherwise known as your VO2 max). This is your body's ability to run at a given pace more efficiently. It should give you faster mile times and more endurance because your body is learning to use less energy while running.
2) Hill work - Love it or hate it, you should be doing it. This style will help you develop power and strength.
3) Long run - This style will help to increase endurance, push your body at a lower intensity for a longer time period, and get your body used to the changes it'll go through on race day. These runs are also good for trying out gear, fuel, hydration and anything else you plan to use on race day.

I recommend adding these three styles after you have a decent base mileage of 15-20 miles per week for a couple solid months.

These workouts are more taxing on your body than a regular run, so you first need a strong foundation.

SPEED WORK

There are different options for speed work. Here are a few types to get you started:
- Interval training - This is running in periods of high intensity for short durations split up by recovery windows. Some interval splits to try are 30/60sec, 1/2min, 90sec/3min. For example, in a 30/60sec split you would work for 30 seconds and recover for 60. Interval training tends to keep the heart rate elevated throughout the workout.
- Repeats - These are similar to interval training, except that they allow full recovery between working phases. In a repeat, you would run a specific distance as hard as you could, then rest until your heart rate recovers so you can hit it again just as hard. Every repeat should match from the first to the last. For example, if you do your first 200m repeat in 45 seconds, your sixth should be 45 seconds. It is common to do 6-8 repeats, but you can go up to 20+ depending on the level of conditioning.

- Fartlek runs - "Fartlek" is Swedish for "speed play," which is exactly what you end up doing. These are typically longer runs over longer distance, but similar to interval training you'll vary your pace as you go.

If you're new to running, you should push for light to medium effort until you build a strong base. As that base grows, incorporate more advanced running days into your plan slowly.

Remember to adjust the workouts based on your athletic level. Ease into higher intensity runs, and make sure to give your body time to recover.

HILL WORKOUTS

Hills, hills, and more hills! Hill training is one style that never seems to end for me. It's a great workout for developing power and strength and prepare your body for those hills on race day.

Remember that running downhill can cause serious stress on your joints. I recommend running up and walking down to recover, unless you're a trail runner and this is specifically part of your training plan.

All you need to run hills is ... well, one hill, or a treadmill that allows for incline adjustment. I do most of my hill work on a treadmill because I don't have any decent hills nearby and my schedule doesn't allow for far travel.

When looking for a hill, think about the type of work you want to do. Two common types are rolling hills and sprinting hills.

- With rolling hills, try to find a stretch of trail or road with gradual rolling hills where you can run a sustained half mile to a mile. You shouldn't be maxing out on every hill, but the workload should feel more intense than running a flat course.
- For hill sprints, try to find a hill with a more aggressive incline. These allow for short duration sprints up the hill, followed by a walk or jog back down depending on the grade (AKA the slope of the hill).

Just like with speed work, you want to have a base mileage before you start upping intensity.

When you do start adjusting your plan, pay special attention to your body. If you have sharp or mild pain that lasts longer than a couple days, get it looked at.

Hill training is a great way to add variation and progress toward that next PR (personal record). As much as some complain about hills, they can be a welcome change if you're getting bored of running the same routes.

LONG RUN

The long run! Everyone's favorite weekend task, I'm sure.

Long runs help for a few reasons, but there are three key benefits: increasing base mileage and endurance, getting closer to simulating race day mileage, and testing any gear/nutrition you have planned for race day.

- Increasing base mileage and endurance - This means you are progressively adding to the number of miles you average in a week. For this to happen safely and efficiently, it needs to be gradual. (Remember the earlier discussion on safe progression.) When adding to your base, stay in zone 2 for the bulk of your miles. It's less taxing on the body and is where you will reap the most benefits to build endurance.

- Getting closer to race day mileage - Simulating what your body will go through on race day is a great way to be physically ready, and it also prepares you mentally. Knowing what your body will feel like in those last two miles can put you at ease during the race, and allows you to better deal with the stress.
- Testing race day gear and nutrition - This third benefit is critical. Test your gear! No new gear on race day! This rule can make or break a race. There should be no surprises from your gear or nutrition outside of a catastrophic failure.
- Trying out race day conditions - If you only go out for mid-day sunshine runs, but race day will start at 7 a.m. in the spring, you might want to try a long run before sunrise.
- Experiment with rain - Splash around in some puddles. See how your shoes and feet handle being wet. I don't recommend this on your first try or early on in a long run (hello, blisters), but it is helpful to know what to expect if it begins raining on race day.

SECTION 4 — RECOVERY & INJURIES

In this section we will discuss the following:
- Recovery techniques
- Dynamic stretching
- Static stretching
- Foam rolling
- R.I.C.E.
- Recovery weeks
- Taper time

RECOVERY TECHNIQUES

Recovery is essential from day one through the rest of your running journey. Don't just think about recovering post-exercise. Think about an overall recovery plan.

This plan should include recovery techniques pre- and post-workout, and activities to promote healing and recovery on both rest days and cross training days.

Here is an overview of recovery techniques, then we'll discuss each one more in-depth:

- Sleep - This is so important for recovery and often overlooked. You need to get enough quality sleep so your body can repair and rebuild.
- Dynamic stretching - Done pre-workout.
- Static stretching - Done post-workout.
- Foam Rolling - Can be done any time to support recovery of sore muscles and connective tissue.
- RICE (Rest, Ice, Compression, and Elevation) - Done after an injury to help recovery.
- Recovery runs & recovery weeks - A technique that uses zone 1 or 2 training to assist in recovery.
- Taper - A period of recovery before a race that allows you to fully recover from training and feel fresh on race day.

The most important thing to remember is that recovery is way more than five minutes of stretching post-workout or a rest day once a week. Recovery is your body repairing and adapting to the stress of training. It is when the real progress is made.

STRETCHING — DYNAMIC

Dynamic stretching should be used before your workout as part of the warmup. This type of stretching is especially helpful before high intensity workouts like speed training or hill work.

Dynamic stretching uses movement to stretch muscles. You don't hold any stretch. It is a fluid, "dynamic" movement.

Dynamic stretching works to warm and prepare your muscles, increase your range of motion, and improve your spatial awareness (being aware of your own body in space). These three benefits translate to better control of your body and will make you less prone to injury.
You do need to be careful when using dynamic stretching. Stay in control of the movement. Too much and you can end up doing more harm than good.

The next level of stretching past dynamic is called ballistic stretching. It uses momentum to push past what a dynamic stretch can provide. I chose not to cover that here because it is very advanced and should only be done under supervision.

The takeaway: We can all benefit from dynamic stretching. Just remember to take things slow and stay in control.

STRETCHING — STATIC

Static (or stationary) stretching should primarily be used post-workout after your cooldown. It improves flexibility and range of motion, and it can help lessen pain and stiffness.

Perform the stretch with some resistance, but never to a point that becomes painful. Never bounce or force a position, which can overextend the muscle and cause injury.

Try to hold the stretch for 30 seconds to a minute while maintaining calm and steady breaths. Don't forget to breathe!
The overall experience should be pleasant and relaxing, while at the same time you should be able to feel the target muscles being stretched. Budget 10-15 minutes post-run for static stretching, and your body will thank you.

This is just the tip of the iceberg for stretching. If you have an area giving you trouble, I encourage you to dive deeper and find ways to target that muscle specifically or check in with a medical professional.

FOAM ROLLING

If you haven't tried this, pay attention! It took me over a year of running before I started foam rolling because I didn't know the many benefits of one simple practice.

Foam rolling can help with tightness, sore muscles, mobility, and can even help underlying issues that cause joint pain.

It works by reducing soreness and tightness in a couple of ways. It increases blood flow to the area post-workout, which then allows delivery of nutrients and removal of waste products.

Foam rolling can also be used pre-workout to help with mobility and flexibility by warming up and loosening the targeted muscles, which then relieves pressure on connective tissue and joints.

There are some precautions to take:

- Avoid joints and connective tissue as foam rolling can put undue stress on the area and potentially cause injury. Muscle is what benefits from this practice, so target the muscles that support the tissue or joint problem area.

- Be cautious with pressure. It shouldn't be excruciatingly painful to get through your foam rolling routine.

- Never foam roll an injury. Doing so will be painful and can exacerbate the problem. If you think you may have an injury, seek medical advice ASAP.

Depending on the areas targeted, foam rolling can take a couple of minutes or 10+ minutes. Plan on about 30 seconds per targeted muscle.

R.I.C.E.

Rest. Ice. Compression. Elevation.
If you have experienced an injury, seek advice from a medical professional. If you have some mild pain that isn't severe enough to warrant a visit, try the RICE method. These four things can help alleviate a lot of pain and speed recovery:
1) REST - Rest the injury. Give your body the time it needs to heal. It likely won't happen overnight, but respect the process. Trying to rush back in too early can have horrible consequences.

2) ICE - Icing the area can temporarily relieve pain and help with swelling and inflammation. Never apply ice directly to the skin as direct exposure can cause frostbite. You can try icing the area for 20 minutes every four hours for the first 48 hours. (Icing more than 20 minutes can result in additional tissue damage.)

3) COMPRESSION - Use an ace bandage to wrap the area. The wrap should be snug to help keep swelling down, but not too tight that it impairs circulation. Loosen the wrap if you feel numbness, tingling, increased pain, coolness, or swelling around the bandage.

4) ELEVATION - Elevate the injury above your heart to let gravity help the healing process. This draws fluids away from the injured area and helps with swelling.

Remember if the injury is significant or doesn't improve in 24-48 hours, consider seeking medical attention.
A minor injury can quickly turn major if left undiagnosed, and a couple weeks of bedrest could turn into a couple months or a whole season.

RECOVERY WEEKS

If you are pushing hard with high-intensity effort or long distances week after week, the increased stress can accumulate over time. Some training programs add recovery weeks to help deal with the slowly accumulated stress.

A recovery week is one with reduced mileage. They are typically laced into a training plan between 2-4 build weeks. An example might look like:

Week 1 – Build: 45 miles
Week 2 – Build: 47 miles
Week 3 – Build: 51 miles
Week 4 – Recovery: 25 miles
Week 5 – Build: 51 miles
Week 6 – Build: 53 miles

The recovery week breaks up the build weeks and lets your body adjust to the increasing mileage. They are usually seen in plans geared to longer duration or base building.

If you are struggling to increase base mileage and keep hitting stalls, consider adding a recovery week to your training plan.

TAPER TIME

At the tail end of your training plan leading up to race day is a length of time called the taper. This is when you should significantly scale back training to let your body heal.

Taper will allow you to take all of your training and convert it into results. The goal is to go into race day 100% charged up and ready to explode.

Although it is a time to recover, these aren't complete rest days. You should be focusing on recovery, staying active, and dialing in your nutrition plan. There should also be some light training during taper to keep your body working. Think zone 2 work.

Taper time can vary depending on the training plan and the event. Usually the more intense the event and training, the longer the taper. If you are running a 5K, you shouldn't need as long a taper as someone running an Ironman.

With a greatly scaled back exercise schedule, you should feel like you have a lot of extra time, so don't waste it. Channel that time into supporting your race effort. Take it seriously.

This is the culmination of weeks or months of training. It deserves just as much, if not more, respect than the entire buildup to this point.

SECTION 5 – PROPER FORM

In this section we will discuss the following:
- Running form overview
- Good posture
- Foot strike
- Cadence & stride
- Rotational & forward movement

RUNNING FORM OVERVIEW

When starting your running journey, the primary objectives should be getting acclimated to running and building a base mileage. Running form at this stage should be geared toward injury prevention over optimization and efficiency gain.

Remember that we are all built differently. While there are generalities that can be widely applied, there are also situations where they cannot.

I would never recommend anyone make drastic changes to their running form based on what is considered "correct" or "proper."

If you choose to apply some of these principles, do so slowly and gradually.

There are many components to running form, so we'll look at an overview then dive into each individually.

- Good posture - This refers to staying tall, centered and stabilizing your core as you run.
- Foot strike - This refers to how your foot strikes the ground.
- Cadence - This is the number of steps you take in a minute.
- Stride length - This is the distance between successive ground contacts of the same foot. Think of it as the measurement of two steps forward.
- Rotational movement – In the context of this book we will refer specifically to your arm swing. Runners can develop a tendency to swing their arms with rotational movement, which is counterproductive.

GOOD POSTURE

Running with good posture can increase running efficiency, open your airway so you can breathe easier, and reduce injuries to your lower back, knees and hips.

To maintain good posture, run "tall." In other words, don't slouch when you're running. You want to be centered and running with a stable core. You can lean slightly into the run, but don't slouch or hunch over.

Running on a treadmill in front of a mirror is a good way to check your form. If you're far off, work slowly to improve your posture.
Drastic changes in form can lead to overusing muscles that may not be as strong as they need to be to deal with the newly added stress.

FOOT STRIKE

The most common foot strike is a rearfoot strike, sometimes called a heel strike. There is also a midfoot strike and a forefoot strike.

The rearfoot strike is the most critiqued form. Here are a couple reasons of thought about it, and additional things to consider.

1) It is inefficient due to the increased braking force, which refers to loss of forward momentum when your heel strikes the ground.

Consider that braking force may not be 100% from the rearfoot strike. It could be caused by over striding, which means your foot is landing too far further out in front. If you're over striding, it will contribute to braking no matter what your foot strike is.

2) It increases impact to joints (like the knee).

Keep in mind that impact is magnified by pace. At a slower pace, the impact will be lower and is less noticeable. Also, when you reach "sprinting" speeds, your body should naturally push into a mid- or forefoot strike to protect the joints.

Before you try adjusting your foot strike, consider these points:

- Changing foot strike is hard to do on a consistent basis, especially if you are still trying to find your rhythm, or your level of conditioning doesn't allow for relaxed runs in which you can focus on foot strike.

- Deliberately changing how your foot lands can sometimes shift the injury from one area to another (knee to calf for example).

- Look at the other aspects of your form. Should you put the time into adjusting your foot strike, or are there other areas you could focus on first like arm swing or cadence? Remember that adjusting form should be done through slow and gradual progress.

CADENCE AND STRIDE

Cadence + stride length = speed. Increase one or the other and you increase your speed. Let's look at both and how they interact.

Cadence is your number of steps per minute. Most average runners are in the 150-170 range, but an ideal range is closer to 180. You can find yours with most smart watches or by counting the number of steps you take in one minute.

Increasing your cadence has several benefits. It will pull your foot strike back and reduce braking inefficiency. It can reduce impact on your joints. And once you're used to a higher cadence, it can lessen the perceived effort and make running more comfortable.

When trying to increase cadence, do so in gradual steps. You can find music at your target cadence by searching for playlists at a certain BPM. These are available on almost all streaming platforms.

Stride length is the second building block of speed. It is measured as the distance between successive ground contacts of the same foot.

For example, start with feet together at Point A. Step forward with your right foot, then take another step with your left. Where your left foot just landed is Point B. Measure between A and B to find your stride length.

When increasing stride length, try to propel farther forward instead of just reaching out farther with each step. If you move your foot strike too far out, you can add unnecessary impact and braking force. Think of it like pulling your heel up into your glute and driving forward with your whole body.

Increasing stride comes from strength and power. To develop both, try incorporating hill workouts into your training plan. (See Section 3 for some cautionary points.)

ROTATIONAL & FORWARD MOVEMENT

Arm swing is an easy area to improve for most new runners. Proper arm swing will keep you running efficiently and will reduce fatigue in your arms and shoulders.

Your arms should be between your waist and chest with elbows bent at roughly a 90-degree angle. Stay loose and try to keep arm movement minimal. You can slightly propel yourself using your arms, but don't go overboard with an exaggerated swing.

Try to use forward movement as much as possible. Don't let your arms swing across your body or side to side. One trick is to pull your elbows in toward your sides.

Arm swing should generate from the shoulder forward and backward. Try to eliminate any up and down movement in the shoulder. This is key to keeping your upper body loose and avoiding tension.

I should note that not all rotational movement is counterproductive to propelling yourself forward.

There are some advanced techniques such as counter-rotation of the spine and engaging the hips to produce power.

However, I find such techniques a bit out of scope for entry-level running. If you are curious, look further into that topic or feel free to reach out to me. I'd be happy to help.

SECTION 6 — READY FOR RACE DAY

In this section we will discuss the following:
- What to expect on race day
- Packet pickup
- Arriving early
- Eating pre-race
- Starting corrals
- Course etiquette

YOU PICKED A RACE! NOW WHAT?

Congratulations! You got the hard part out of the way. Now just keep training in preparation for the big day.

I've included here information and tips to help put your mind at ease before a first race.

First, let's look at an overview of race day, and then we'll look at some aspects more in depth.

- 1-2 days before – The lead up to race day is when the experience starts. You'll have 48 hours to get ready physically, mentally, and emotionally. You should be in your taper at this point.
- 3-4 hours before – This is when to eat your pre-race meal.
- Arrive early – Plan to get there at least an hour early.
- Packet pickup – Grab your race packet, which includes your bib and any promotional items (food or beer tickets, ads, etc.).
- Last minute bathroom break – Be ready for long lines and wait times depending on the size of the race.
- Stretching and warmup – It's easy to get caught up in the race day festival atmosphere, but don't forget this is a race. You need to stretch and warm up. You're here to run after all!
- Lining up in the starting corrals – Line up and get ready for that countdown!
- Post-race – Time for the party! Get your medal at the finish line and throw it on. Grab some food and a beverage and relax. You earned it!

PACKET PICKUP

This is one of those things that might be intimidating for a first race. Don't worry though; it's no big deal.

Packet pickup is just you grabbing your race day packet of information prior to the race.

Find out ahead of time when packet pickup is, if they offer an early pickup, or have mandatory packet pickup that does not fall on race day.

Make sure you choose the right line. Nothing is more frustrating than standing in line for "packet pickup" to realize you're in the line for same day registration.

The workers will likely need to scan your barcode from the race registration and check your license, so bring both.

It's easy to pull up the registration email on your phone, but I like to download and print the email just in case. Depending on the size of the race, you and possibly thousands of others are there and cell service might be an issue.

Depending on the event, you may be able to grab packets for any family members racing with you - I have grabbed my wife's before.

Included in your race day packet will be your race bib (this gets pinned to your clothing), probably any food or drink tickets, and likely some advertising flyers.

Some races have bib pins on the table - make sure you grab four per bib. Or, if you want to skip the safety pins, you can find affordable racing bib pins online.

ARRIVING EARLY

I can't say this enough. Make sure you arrive early. This will help your anxiety more than almost anything else you can do.

At a minimum, get there an hour early. If it's your first race and you're going solo or with other first timers, I would recommend an extra half hour so you can explore, get lost, run back to the car because you forgot something..., etc.

Think about the line of cars that might be waiting to get into the event. I have seen hour-long waits one mile from the venue.

You don't want to be scrambling to get to the starting line at the expense of skipping a warmup or getting caught in the bathroom line. If you have stuck to a consistent training schedule, now is not the time to fall behind. Give yourself plenty of time, and you'll be thankful.

EATING PRE-RACE

We have looked at pre-run, intra-run, and post-run nutrition, but I want to talk about eating pre-race and the days leading up to it.

By race week you should know exactly what you are going to eat for at least 24 hours before. This will limit the likelihood of digestive issues derailing a PR.

Follow these three rules and you should be able to finish your race with no digestive issues.

First Rule – NOTHING NEW ON RACE DAY.
The food you eat should be food you have already tried prior to running. Have a couple practice runs weeks before. Log what you eat before long runs a few weeks in a row and compare that to how your run felt.

Second Rule – Carb load properly.
Based on your long run experiments, you may decide to carb load with your pre-race meal. This should consist of a slightly higher carb count than a pre-run meal in order to top off your glycogen.

Remember that glycogen stores are limited. Once they're full, your body starts storing what it can as fat and getting rid of the rest. So don't binge on pasta and bread, or be prepared for some digestive issues.

Third Rule – Don't forget electrolytes.
Begin focusing on hydration a few days prior to the event, not the night before. Refer to Section 2 for more information on hydration.

STARTING CORRALS

It's your first race day, you have your bib on, warmup is complete, bathroom needs are met, and you're walking to the starting corral...

This feeling of jittery nervousness is very short lived because once that race starts everything fades away. You're doing exactly what you've done so many times before - just running.

Soak it in because this feeling is what will push you to sign up for another race as soon as you cross the finish line.

There are a few things to pay attention to when it comes to lining up at the start line.

Find out whether your race is conducted in heats or if it's the same start time for all runners. If the race is in heats, you'll need to line up for your specific heat.

You generally won't be able to jump ahead, but most races will accommodate runners who miss their heat and need to jump into a later one. Check the details for your specific race.

If the race starts in one big group, then it may be split by pace times depending on the number of runners. If you see pace times along the corral barricades, then find the section of the corral marked for your estimated pace.

If there are no pace times or guidance, then it is usually faster runners up front and those with a more casual pace toward the back.

I've had many people try to push past me to get to the front, and I let these people breeze by.

It can get a little packed in the beginning, but after the first half mile the pack will thin out. Be patient.

COURSE ETIQUETTE

You're out of the corral! Now let's look at some common things you'll see on the course.

- Passing - When it comes to pace and passing, the general rule is slower runners stay to the right and passing is done on the left. It is also common to call out "on your left" when passing, but during a race with many runners this isn't as feasible.
When passing, make sure you have enough in the tank to maintain your passing pace. There is nothing more frustrating than someone passing you only to slow down 30 seconds later and break your pace.

- Water stations - These can be a bit intense. If you can't drink on the go then grab your cup, move past the station and stop near the side of the course. Don't stop in front of the station and jam it up.

- It is usually acceptable to toss the cups directly after the water station (race volunteers pick these up). THIS DOESN'T APPLY ELSEWHERE. Don't litter. If you generate trash on course, find a trash can or take it back out with you.

- Spitting and clearing your nose - These are very common on course, but any time you're running with others, do everyone a favor and check behind you before letting loose.

Overall just be the person you'd want to meet. Race employees, volunteers, spectators, and fellow racers are all there to have a good time (most of them anyhow). If everyone tries even a little bit to improve the experience for others, we all have a great time.

SECTION 7 — BONUS MATERIAL

In this section we will discuss the following:
- Dealing with the weather < 45 degrees
- Dealing with the weather > 45 degrees
- How to avoid boredom on runs
- Aerobic vs anaerobic exercises
- Benefits of adding strength training

DEALING WITH THE WEATHER
< 45 DEGREES

Dressing for the weather can make or break a run and when it comes to extremes it can be downright dangerous to be unprepared. Wind, rain, snow, sun, and everything in between carries with its different requirements.

We'll start with cold temperatures and work our way up. (All temperatures are in Fahrenheit.)

In cold temperatures it may not feel like you're sweating, but you still need to hydrate. It's easy to overlook dehydration in the cold because you aren't as hot and sweaty as you get in warmer weather.

Watch out for ice! Running on fresh snow is no problem but temperatures that swing above and below freezing pose a significant risk of black ice, which can be bad news!

< 10 degrees – These temperatures can be downright dangerous. If you plan to go out in single digits or below, you should be in three or more layers and have no skin exposed. Exposed skin risks frostbite, which doesn't take long at these temperatures.

10-32 degrees – These temperatures are a little more manageable but still carry the risk of frostbite. At the upper end you can probably drop down to two layers instead of three, and you might be able to drop to lighter gloves.

32-45 degrees – You are entering more bearable temperatures, and some early and late season races will see these temps for an early morning start. If this is morning temp think two layers that you can peel off or vent easily as the day warms. A scarf is my personal preference especially if there is a stiff wind.

DEALING WITH THE WEATHER
> 45 DEGREES

Now things are warming up.

45-60 degrees – The perfect zone for most. You won't be drenched in sweat, and you don't have to worry about cold weather gear at the mid and upper end.

60-80 degrees – Things are starting to get hot on the run. At the upper end you'll have to start focusing more on hydration.

80-95 degrees – Don't forget your water bottle. Stay safe and stay hydrated.

> 95 degrees – Proceed with caution. Hydration will be an issue and watch for signs of heat exhaustion and heat stroke. Listen to your body.

Precipitation isn't as big a deal above 45 degrees and can help to cool you off. It does make things a little slick though, and trail runners may also have mud to deal with.

I would never recommend running through a thunderstorm. Some may say the risk of lightning is low, but I consider it a risk not worth taking.

High wind can be a bit of a P.I.T.A., but you can also view it as extra resistance training.

Overall, stay mindful of the weather. A recurring theme with running is preparation and when it comes to the elements, preparation and planning are king.

Dress appropriately and you'll be fine. Don't take it seriously and you'll have a miserable run (or worse you might get a very expensive ride to the hospital).

HOW TO AVOID BOREDOM ON RUNS

It's funny how many people I talk to who will say, "I could never be a runner; I get so bored!"

I cringe a little when I hear that. How many times do you catch yourself saying, "I just wish I had a little more me time"?

Wouldn't it be great if that time was also lowering your stress, helping you manage your weight, and increasing your physical fitness?

Hello, running!

Here are my favorite ways to avoid boredom:

- Podcasts – Podcasts can make the time FLY by, and most are free. Find one you like and zone out.
- Audio Books – Have a book you want to read, but no time to read it? Audio books are a great way to pass time on a casual jog.
- Pace Counting – This works for some and not for others. I find that counting my pace in sets of 2 or 4 helps get through a few miles and also helps with breathing. Make a game out of it and see how high you can get without losing count.
- Get Outside – A nice nature trail provides plenty of sights and sounds to distract you.
- Music – The obvious one. I run a lot so my favorites aren't favorites for long. What I've done is built one big playlist with all kinds of music. When a certain song or genre hits the spot, I take 2 seconds to start a radio station off that song. Variety is key here.
- Movies and Shows – Treadmill running is boring. No getting around it. Try playing a movie or a show next time you're on the treadmill and see if it helps pass the time.

AEROBIC VS ANAEROBIC EXERCISE

Let's look at the difference between aerobic and anaerobic exercises and how it plays into running.

Aerobic means relating to, involving, or requiring free oxygen. In an aerobic state your body has an adequate supply of oxygen. You can sustain this pace for long periods of time.

It also means your body is utilizing fat as a primary energy source because it has enough oxygen to process the fat, and waste is generated at a level your body can keep up with.

Anaerobic is the opposite. Your body is working in an oxygen deficiency. When you cross this threshold, your body is no longer getting enough oxygen to utilize fat as a primary fuel source, so it taps into stored glycogen.

Using glycogen and generating energy at an accelerated rate will generate waste at a rate that your body can no longer keep up with.

(Keep in mind your body is almost always using both sources of fuel in both states; it's the percentages of each that are changing).

Pay attention on your next run and see if you can feel the difference between the two stages.

BENEFITS OF ADDING STRENGTH TRAINING

Strength training is often overlooked by new runners, but I recommend incorporating it throughout your running career. It is just too beneficial to pass up.

Running conditions your body for the miles it will endure, but strength training can improve your speed and efficiency, lower injury potential, and improve your overall fitness level.

When considering strength training, don't just think about the major muscles that support running. It should be a balanced plan that targets lower body, upper body, and core.

Start with two to three days per week added to your training plan.

If you don't have access to a gym, try a bodyweight exercise. I have one available for free download here: https://endurance-athletics.com/downloads/

Don't neglect core work. There is a lot going on when you run, and a lot of it gets channeled through your core.

You also have a lot of stabilizing muscles that tie in through the back and core. Show these some extra love and attention, because they're what you'll use to step up near the end of a run when you start to fatigue.

Injury can creep in when you reach fatigue, so have these muscles conditioned and up for the challenge to stay ahead of the game.

END NOTES

That's it! If you made it this far, I appreciate you taking the time to read through my book.

I hope you got something useful out of it.

Remember everyone has a Day 1. We all started out brand new at some point.

It is truly my hope that this book helps someone who is hesitant to pick up running.

It can be such an amazing way to improve yourself physically and mentally.

Follow me on Instagram @matthofbauer_ to get information on upcoming projects including:

- Nutrition For Runners - An in-depth look at how to support your running through proper nutrition.
- Running Terminology – A reference sheet for all the crazy terms and abbreviations that we use in the running community.

Feel free to reach out through a DM on Instagram or through my contact page at
https://endurance-athletics.com/contact/

Thank you so much for reading.
Stay safe out there!

Printed in Great Britain
by Amazon